HUNTINGTON'S DISEASE MANAGEMENT DIET COOKBOOK

I0477798

Nutritional Strategies For Wellness: A

Guide To Holistic Care: Recipes For

Health: Nourish Your Body, Empower

Your Journey

DR. SHAYLA LEWIS

Table of Contents

DISCLAIMER

Write a brief complete Disclaimer for my diet cook book telling them that the author is not in any association with any company, business or individual and also this book is written by the authors knowledge and understanding

The information provided in this diet cookbook is based on the author's personal knowledge and understanding. The author is not affiliated with, endorsed by, or associated with any company, business, or individual. The recipes and dietary advice contained within this book are intended for informational purposes only. Readers should consult with a healthcare professional or a registered dietitian before making any significant changes to their diet or lifestyle. The author assumes no responsibility for any adverse effects that may result from the use or misuse of the information contained in this book.

CHAPTER ONE

Understanding Huntington's Disease and Its Impact: Huntington's disease is a neurodegenerative ailment that destroys nerve cells in the brain over time, causing gradual physical, cognitive, and emotional loss. It can lead to uncontrollable movements, cognitive impairment, and mental disorders. Understanding the disease's course and impact on daily living is critical for effective symptom management and sustaining quality of life.

Nutrition is important in managing Huntington's disease since it can have an impact on general health and well-being.

A well-balanced, nutrient-dense diet can promote cognitive function, preserve muscular mass, and boost energy levels. A proper diet can also help alleviate some symptoms and decrease the progression of the disease, making it an important component of holistic care for Huntington's patients.

Low-carb, antioxidant-rich, and anti-inflammatory diets can help people with Huntington's disease. These dietary approaches primarily aim to reduce inflammation in the body, which is thought to contribute to disease progression. Antioxidant-rich foods like fruits, vegetables, nuts, and seeds can help protect brain cells from harm. Furthermore, limiting carbohydrate intake can assist to stabilise blood sugar levels and enhance general health.

How This Cookbook Can Help You:

This cookbook is specifically developed for those living with Huntington's disease, providing a collection of dishes adapted to their dietary needs and preferences. Each dish is meticulously designed to be low in carbohydrates, high in antioxidants, and anti-inflammatory, resulting in both delicious meals and therapeutic advantages. This cookbook, with simple directions and readily available materials, aims to simplify meal preparation and assist persons in keeping a balanced diet despite disease problems.

Tips for Getting Started with the Recipes: Using the recipes in this cookbook is simple and uncomplicated. Begin by becoming familiar with the ingredients and equipment required for each recipe.

Plan your meals ahead of time so you have all of the supplies on hand. Begin with one or two recipes that appeal to you, then gradually extend your repertoire as you gain confidence in the kitchen. Don't be afraid to experiment and make changes to suit your taste and dietary requirements. Most importantly, enjoy the process of cooking and providing your body with great, nutritious meals.

Huntington's disease has a major impact on everyday functioning and overall quality of life for both patients and carers. Basic actions like walking, eating, and conversing become more difficult as the condition develops. Maintaining independence and quality of life takes thoughtful planning and assistance.

Nutrition is essential for treating symptoms and reducing the progression of Huntington's disease.

A well-balanced diet high in antioxidants, omega-3 fatty acids, and vitamins can improve brain function and reduce inflammation. Proper nutrition can also help with symptoms including weight loss and swallowing issues, which improves overall health.

Common Challenges for Patients and Carers: When dealing with Huntington's Disease, patients and carers confront a variety of challenges, including physical limits, mental stress, and financial pressure. Coping with the disease's progressive nature and adapting to shifting care requirements can be difficult. Seeking help from healthcare professionals and support groups is critical for navigating these problems successfully.

Support and Information Resources: Huntington's Disease patients can find a variety of resources to help them cope with their condition. These include neurology and genetic counseling specialists and advocacy groups. Accessing accurate information and interacting with individuals facing similar issues can provide vital support and direction throughout your Huntington's disease journey.

CHAPTER TWO

Overview of Huntington's Disease and its Symptoms: Huntington's disease is a neurological ailment that causes progressive physical, cognitive, and emotional impairment. Symptoms often appear in maturity and include uncontrollable movements, cognitive impairment, and psychiatric disorders. Understanding these signs is critical for early diagnosis and efficient treatment.

Huntington's disease has a major impact on everyday functioning and overall quality of life for both patients and carers. Basic actions like walking, eating, and conversing become more difficult as the condition develops. Maintaining independence and quality of life takes thoughtful planning and assistance.

Nutrition is essential for treating symptoms and reducing the progression of Huntington's disease. A well-balanced diet high in antioxidants, omega-3 fatty acids, and vitamins can improve brain function and reduce inflammation. Proper nutrition can also help with symptoms including weight loss and swallowing issues, which improves overall health.

Common Challenges for Patients and Carers: When dealing with Huntington's Disease, patients and carers confront a variety of challenges, including physical limits, mental stress, and financial pressure. Coping with the disease's progressive nature and adapting to shifting care requirements can be difficult. Seeking help from healthcare professionals and support groups is critical for navigating these problems successfully.

Support and Information Resources: Huntington's Disease patients can find a variety of resources to help them cope with their condition. These include neurology and genetic counseling specialists, advocacy groups, and online forums. Accessing accurate information and interacting with individuals facing similar issues can provide vital support and direction throughout your Huntington's disease journey.

Understanding the Basics of Low-Carb Diets: Low-carb diets involve eating fewer carbohydrates and more fats and proteins. The idea is to consume full meals such as meat, fish, eggs, veggies, and healthy fats while avoiding processed grains, sweets, and starchy carbohydrates. Understanding the concepts of low-carb diets allows you to make informed decisions about what to eat and what to avoid, ultimately helping you manage Huntington's disease.

Exploring Low-Carb Alternatives to High-Carb Foods: Instead of classic high-carb foods such as pasta, bread, and rice, look into low-carb alternatives that will satisfy your appetites while keeping your carb intake under control. Cauliflower rice or zucchini noodles, for example, can be substituted for rice or pasta in your favorite dishes, while lettuce wraps can be used in place of tortillas or bread. You can enjoy familiar flavors while being low-carb by being creative with alternatives.

Tips for Managing Blood Sugar Levels: Managing blood sugar levels is critical for people with Huntington's disease since fluctuations can affect symptoms and general health. To keep blood sugar constant, consume regular meals and snacks that contain protein, healthy fats, and fiber-rich carbohydrates. Avoid sugary drinks and snacks in favor of water, herbal tea, or unsweetened liquids. Regularly monitoring your blood sugar levels can also help you understand how different foods affect you and make necessary modifications.

Delicious Low-Carb Recipes for Every Meal: Try a variety of low-carb recipes to keep your meals interesting and rewarding. Start your day with a veggie-packed omelette or a smoothie containing leafy greens and protein powder. For lunch, try a robust salad with lots of protein and avocado for healthy fats. Dinner alternatives can include grilled salmon with roasted veggies or a stir-fry with tofu and low-carb vegetables. Don't forget about snacks—nuts, cheese, and vegetables with hummus are great options for keeping you going between meals.

How to Stay Satisfied and Energised on a Low-Carb Diet: Maintaining a low-carb diet requires balance and variety. To stay full and satisfied, make sure each meal has a combination of protein, healthy fats, and non-starchy vegetables. Experiment with new flavors' and cuisines to keep your taste buds happy, and don't be afraid to include occasional sweets or high-carb meals in moderation. Maintain hydration, get enough of sleep, and prioritise stress management to improve your overall health while following a low-carb diet for Huntington's disease treatment.

CHAPTER THREE
Cooking Methods for Healthier Meals
Healthy Cooking Techniques for Huntington's Disease Management

Use steaming, baking, grilling, and sautéing with little oil to produce meals that retain nutrients while reducing bad fats. These strategies aid in the preservation of vitamins and minerals, which are critical for individuals managing Huntington's Disease. Steam veggies to preserve vitamins, or bake fish with herbs instead of frying.

Tips to Reduce Fat and Sodium in Recipes

Instead of using salt, replace butter with olive or avocado oil and add herbs, spices, and citrus juices to enhance the flavours. For example, in sauces, replace heavy cream with Greek yoghurt, and season foods with garlic, lemon, and basil to avoid adding sodium. Choose low-sodium broths and rinse canned vegetables to limit sodium intake.

Maximising flavour without sacrificing health benefits.

Use fresh herbs, spices, citrus zests, and infused vinegars to organically enhance the flavour of your food. For example, marinade chicken in lemon juice, rosemary, and garlic before grilling, or put cinnamon and nutmeg on roasted sweet potatoes for a flavour boost. These ingredients improve taste while also promoting a healthy diet.

Kitchen Tools & Gadgets that Simplify Meal Prep

Invest in a slow cooker, a food processor, and a set of sharp knives to make meal preparation easier and quicker. A slow cooker may help you make nutritious soups and stews with little effort, and a food processor can rapidly chop vegetables or combine smoothies. Sharp knives ensure precise and safe cutting, which reduces prep time.

Cooking Tips for Busy Days and On-The-Go Meals

To save time on hectic days, prepare and portion meals ahead of time. Ingredients such as cereals, meats, and vegetables can be batch cooked and refrigerated for easy assembly into balanced meals. Use mason jars to store layered salads or overnight oats, ensuring that nutritional options are readily available when needed. Freeze smoothie packs for quick breakfasts.

The Importance of a Healthy Breakfast for Huntington's Disease Management

A healthy breakfast is essential for controlling Huntington's disease since it helps to stabilise energy levels and improves cognitive performance throughout the day. Whole grains, lean proteins, and healthy fats help improve brain function and provide long-lasting energy. For example, starting your day with a bowl of muesli topped with berries and almonds, or a vegetable omelette with whole-grain bread, can provide critical nutrients that help with symptom management and overall well-being.

Quick and Simple Breakfast Ideas for Busy Mornings

On busy mornings, choose simple and quick breakfast options that do not skimp on nutrition. A smoothie made with spinach, banana, almond milk, and a scoop of protein powder takes only a few minutes to make and is loaded with vitamins and minerals. Alternatively, create overnight oats the night before by combining oats, chia seeds, almond milk, and honey in a jar for a quick and nutritious breakfast.

Recipes for energising smoothies and protein-rich breakfasts

Energising smoothies and protein-rich meals are ideal for keeping your energy levels and muscles healthy. Make a smoothie with Greek yoghurt, frozen berries, spinach, and a tablespoon of flaxseeds for a nutrient-dense start to the day. For a protein-rich breakfast, try a quinoa breakfast bowl with sautéed vegetables and a poached egg, or a tofu scramble with bell peppers, onions, and turmeric for an anti-inflammatory boost.

Delicious low-carb options that will keep you satisfied until lunch.

Low-carb breakfast options can help regulate blood sugar levels and alleviate the mid-morning slump.

Try a vegetable frittata with eggs, spinach, mushrooms, and cheese that can be prepared ahead of time and reheated. Another choice is avocado toast on low-carb bread with cherry tomatoes and a drizzle of olive oil, which has good fats and fibre to keep you full and content until lunchtime.

CHAPTER FOUR

Tips for preparing breakfasts ahead of time for convenience.

Preparing breakfasts ahead of time can save you time in the morning while providing a nutritious start to your day. Make egg muffins by mixing eggs with chopped vegetables and baking in a muffin tin for a quick, portable breakfast. Overnight chia pudding, produced by soaking chia seeds in almond milk with honey and vanilla, can be made the night before and served with your favourite toppings such as fruit and nuts for a quick, ready-to-eat meal.

Developing Balanced Meals for Huntington's Disease Management

To create balanced meals that help control Huntington's disease, combine lean proteins, healthy fats, and complex carbohydrates in each dish. For example, grilled chicken breast with quinoa and veggie salad contains a healthy balance of protein, fibre, and important elements. Including healthy fats such as avocado or olive oil can improve nutrient absorption and provide anti-inflammatory properties. Remember to incorporate a variety of colourful veggies to guarantee a diverse intake of vitamins and minerals.

Delicious Salad Recipes with Nutrient-Rich Ingredients

Creating excellent salads with nutrient-dense ingredients is both simple and delightful. Begin with a bed of dark leafy greens like spinach or kale, which are high in antioxidants and fibre.

Include a range of colourful veggies, such as bell peppers, carrots, and tomatoes, for vitamins and texture. Lean proteins, such as grilled salmon or chickpeas, can help you feel full and maintain your muscles. Top with seeds or nuts for healthy fats and texture, then drizzle with a little vinaigrette prepared of olive oil and lemon juice to bring all of the flavours together.

Hearty soups and stews for comfort and nutrition.

Hearty soups and stews are ideal for offering both comfort and nutrition in one pot. Begin with a broth base (chicken, beef, or vegetable) and then add a variety of chopped vegetables such as carrots, celery, and potatoes for fibre and vitamins.

Include some protein, such as beans, lentils, or lean meats like turkey or chicken. Season with herbs and spices like garlic, thyme, and bay leaves to boost flavour without adding calories. Allow the stew to boil until all of the ingredients are cooked and the flavours have melded together, resulting in a nutritious and enjoyable supper.

Satisfying Entrees with Lean Proteins and Whole Grains

Consider meals such as baked salmon with brown rice and steamed broccoli for creating delicious entrées with lean proteins and complete grains. Begin by seasoning the salmon with herbs and lemon, and then bake until cooked. Cook brown rice according per package instructions, leaving a slight chew for texture.

Serve with a large amount of steamed broccoli, lightly seasoned with salt and pepper. This combination gives a well-balanced meal high in protein, fibre, and important nutrients, which promotes overall health and energy.

Tips for Portion Control and Mindful Eating during Lunch and Dinner

Portion control and mindful eating at lunch and dinner need numerous practical strategies. Use smaller plates to visibly regulate portion sizes. Fill half your plate with veggies, one-quarter with lean protein, and the rest with nutritious carbohydrates. To avoid overeating, eat carefully and savour each bite while paying attention to your body's hunger cues. Keeping a meal diary can also assist track portions and identify any behaviours that need to be changed. These activities promote healthier digestion and alleviate the discomfort that can come with overeating.

The Importance of Nutritional Snacks for Managing Hunger and Cravings

Nutritious snacks help people with Huntington's Disease manage their hunger and desires by keeping them energised and supplying necessary nutrients. Choose snacks high in protein, fibre, and healthy fats to keep you full for longer. Greek yoghurt with berries, nuts, and veggie sticks with hummus are some examples. These solutions help to stabilise blood sugar levels, prevent overeating during main meals, and promote general health.

Quick and easy snack ideas for any time of day.

Consider keeping a selection of easy-to-prepare snacks on hand. Sliced fruits, pre-cut vegetables, cheese sticks, and whole-grain crackers are ideal for rapid snacking. Hard-boiled eggs, compact packets of mixed nuts, and single-serving nut butter all make excellent portable options. These snacks need no preparation and are great for busy days or when hunger hits suddenly.

Recipes for homemade trail mix and energy bites.

Making your own trail mixes and energy bites is an enjoyable and customisable approach to ensure healthy snacking. For trail mix, add nuts, seeds, dried fruits, and a small amount of dark chocolate or coconut flakes. For energy bites, combine oats, nut butter, honey, and optional ingredients such as chia seeds, dried fruits, or micro chocolate chips, then roll into bite-size balls. Place in the refrigerator for a quick, nutritious snack that is available anytime you are.

Delicious Side Dishes that Complete Any Meal

Enhance your meals with delectable and nutritious side dishes. Roasted veggies, such as Brussels sprouts, carrots, and sweet potatoes, are simple to cook and packed with nutrients. A quinoa salad with chopped vegetables and a light vinaigrette is an excellent addition. Steamed broccoli with lemon zest, or a fresh cucumber and tomato salad with herbs, can lend a refreshing twist to any main meal.

Smart Swaps for Healthier Snack Options

Making wise substitutions can greatly boost the nutritional value of your snacks. Replace chips with air-popped popcorn or kale chips, and go for entire fruits instead of drinks or sugary treats. Replace sugary granola bars with homemade versions made from oats, nuts, and dried fruits. These easy changes can minimise added sugars and harmful fats while increasing fibre and nutrient intake, resulting in improved overall health.

The Importance of Nutritional Snacks for Managing Hunger and Cravings

Nutritious snacks help people with Huntington's Disease manage their hunger and desires by keeping them energised and supplying necessary nutrients. Choose snacks high in protein, fibre, and healthy fats to keep you full for longer. Greek yoghurt with berries, nuts, and veggie sticks with hummus are some examples. These solutions help to stabilise blood sugar levels, prevent overeating during main meals, and promote general health.

CHAPTER FIVE

Quick and easy snack ideas for any time of day.

Consider keeping a selection of easy-to-prepare snacks on hand. Sliced fruits, pre-cut vegetables, cheese sticks, and whole-grain crackers are ideal for rapid snacking. Hard-boiled eggs, compact packets of mixed nuts, and single-serving nut butter all make excellent portable options. These snacks need no preparation and are great for busy days or when hunger hits suddenly.

Recipes for homemade trail mix and energy bites.

Making your own trail mixes and energy bites is an enjoyable and customisable approach to ensure healthy snacking. For trail mix, add nuts, seeds, dried fruits, and a small amount of dark chocolate or coconut flakes. For energy bites, combine oats, nut butter, honey, and optional ingredients such as chia seeds, dried fruits, or micro chocolate chips, then roll into bite-size balls. Place in the refrigerator for a quick, nutritious snack that is available anytime you are.

Delicious Side Dishes that Complete Any Meal

Enhance your meals with delectable and nutritious side dishes. Roasted veggies, such as Brussels sprouts, carrots, and sweet potatoes, are simple to cook and packed with nutrients.

A quinoa salad with chopped vegetables and a light vinaigrette is an excellent addition. Steamed broccoli with lemon zest, or a fresh cucumber and tomato salad with herbs, can lend a refreshing twist to any main meal.

Smart Swaps for Healthier Snack Options

Making wise substitutions can greatly boost the nutritional value of your snacks. Replace chips with air-popped popcorn or kale chips, and go for entire fruits instead of drinks or sugary treats. Replace sugary granola bars with homemade versions made from oats, nuts, and dried fruits. These easy changes can minimise added sugars and harmful fats while increasing fibre and nutrient intake, resulting in improved overall health.

10 Effective Recipes for Huntington's Disease Management

Salmon & Quinoa Bowl

Ingredients:

One cup quinoa.

Two salmon fillets.

One sliced avocado.

One cup of steamed broccoli.

Combine olive oil, salt, and pepper.

Instructions:

Cook the quinoa according to the package instructions.

Season the salmon with salt and pepper, then bake at 375°F for 15-20 minutes.

Assemble the bowl with quinoa, salmon, avocado, and steamed broccoli. Drizzle with olive oil.

Spinach and Feta Stuffed Chicken Breasts

Ingredients:

Four chicken breasts.

Chop 1 cup of spinach.

Add 1/2 cup feta cheese.

Mince 2 cloves of garlic.

Combine olive oil, salt, and pepper.

Instructions:

Preheat the oven to 375° F.

Combine spinach, feta, and garlic. Cut a pocket in each chicken breast and fill with the mixture.

Season with salt and pepper, then bake for 25-30 minutes.

Blueberry Almond Smoothie

Ingredients:

One cup of blueberries.

One banana.

1 cup almond milk.

One tablespoon almond butter.

1 tablespoon chia seeds

Instructions:

Combine all ingredients and blend until smooth.

Serve immediately.

Lentil and Vegetable Soup

Ingredients:

One cup lentils.

One sliced carrot.

One sliced celery stalk.

One chopped onion.

Mince 2 cloves of garlic.

Four cups of veggie broth.

One can of diced tomatoes.

Instructions:

Sauté the onion, garlic, carrot, and celery in olive oil.

Combine lentils, broth, and tomatoes. Simmer for 30–40 minutes.

Chia Pudding With Berries

Ingredients:

1/4 cup of chia seeds.

One cup of coconut milk.

1 tbsp honey.

1 cup mixed berries.

Instructions:

Mix chia seeds, coconut milk, and honey. Refrigerate overnight.

Before serving, top with a combination of berries.

Sweet potato and black bean tacos.

Ingredients:

Dice two sweet potatoes.

One can of drained black beans

One sliced avocado.

Use 1/2 cup salsa.

Corn tortillas

Instructions:

Roast the sweet potatoes at 400°F for 25 minutes.

Warm tortillas, then fill with sweet potatoes, black beans, avocado, and salsa.

Greek Yoghurt & Berry Parfait

Ingredients:

One cup of Greek yoghurt.

1 cup mixed berries.

Add 1/4 cup granola.

1 tbsp honey.

Instructions:

Layer yoghurt, berries, and granola in a glass.

Drizzle with honey.

Whole Grain Vegetable Stir-Fry

Ingredients:

Two cups of brown rice.

One sliced bell pepper.

One cup of snap peas.

One sliced carrot.

1/2 cup chopped mushrooms

Combine soy sauce and sesame oil.

Instructions:

Cook brown rice according to the package instructions.

Stir-fry the vegetables in sesame oil. Add soy sauce to taste.

Serve with brown rice.

Baked Apple Slices with Cinnamon

Ingredients:

4 sliced apples.

1 tbsp cinnamon.

1 tbsp honey.

1/4 cup chopped walnuts

Instructions:

Preheat the oven to 375° F.

Combine apple slices with cinnamon and honey. Bake for 25 minutes.

Before serving, top with walnuts.

10. Avocado & Tomato Salad

Ingredients:

Dice two avocados.

Dice two tomatoes.

1/2 finely sliced red onion.

1 tablespoon olive oil.

One tablespoon of lemon juice.

Add salt and pepper.

Instructions:

Combine all ingredients in a bowl.

Serve immediately.

30 Day Meal Plan for Huntington's Disease
Week 1:

Day 1:

Breakfast: Greek yoghurt and berry parfait.

Lunch: Spinach and Feta Stuffed Chicken
Breast.

Dinner: Lentil and vegetable soup.

Day 2:

Breakfast: Blueberry almond smoothie.

Lunch: Sweet potato and black bean tacos.

Dinner: Whole grain vegetable stir-fry.

Day 3:

Breakfast: Chia Pudding and Berries.

Lunch: Avocado and tomato salad.

Dinner: Salmon and Quinoa Bowl.

Day 4:

Breakfast: Greek yoghurt and berry parfait.

Lunch: Spinach and Feta Stuffed Chicken Breast.

Dinner: Lentil and vegetable soup.

Day 5:

Breakfast: Blueberry almond smoothie.

Lunch: Sweet potato and black bean tacos.

Dinner: Whole grain vegetable stir-fry.

Day 6:

Breakfast: Chia Pudding and Berries.

Lunch: Avocado and tomato salad.

Dinner: Salmon and Quinoa Bowl.

Day 7:

Breakfast: Greek yoghurt and berry parfait.

Lunch: Spinach and Feta Stuffed Chicken Breast.

Dinner: Lentil and vegetable soup.

Week 2:

Repeat Week 1 with small adjustments, such as using different vegetables or fruits in the meals.

Week 3:

Day 15:

Breakfast: Greek yoghurt and berry parfait.

Lunch: Spinach and Feta Stuffed Chicken Breast.

Dinner: Lentil and vegetable soup.

Day 16:

Breakfast: Blueberry almond smoothie.

Lunch: Sweet potato and black bean tacos.

Dinner: Whole grain vegetable stir-fry.

Day 17:

Breakfast: Chia Pudding and Berries.

Lunch: Avocado and tomato salad.

Dinner: Salmon and Quinoa Bowl.

Day 18:

Breakfast: Greek yoghurt and berry parfait.

Lunch: Spinach and Feta Stuffed Chicken Breast.

Dinner: Lentil and vegetable soup.

Day 19:

Breakfast: Blueberry almond smoothie.

Lunch: Sweet potato and black bean tacos.

Dinner: Whole grain vegetable stir-fry.

Day 20:

Breakfast: Chia Pudding and Berries.

Lunch: Avocado and tomato salad.

Dinner: Salmon and Quinoa Bowl.

Day 21:

Breakfast: Greek yoghurt and berry parfait.

Lunch: Spinach and Feta Stuffed Chicken Breast.

Dinner: Lentil and vegetable soup.

Week 4:

Adjust Week 3 to incorporate diverse whole grains, lean meats, and nutrient-dense vegetables.

Notes:

Stay hydrated by drinking plenty of water and herbal tea.

Snack on nuts, seeds, and fresh fruit in between meals as needed.

Adjust portions for individual needs and activity levels.

Work with a healthcare physician or dietician to customise the plan for unique dietary needs.

Conclusion

Managing Huntington's Disease is a difficult task, but food is critical to enhancing the quality of life for people affected. The recipes and meal plans in this cookbook are intended to be more than just nutritional advice; they are a tool to help patients and their families take control of their health via mindful eating.

Nutrition cannot cure Huntington's disease, but it can dramatically reduce symptoms and promote general health. The emphasis on balanced meals high in antioxidants, omega-3 fatty acids, fibre, and important vitamins and minerals is intended to promote brain health, increase energy levels, and improve muscle performance. Incorporating these nutrient-dense foods into your regular diet will help you manage your weight, retain muscle mass, and avoid secondary health problems like cardiovascular disease and diabetes.

The recipes in this book focus on simplicity and diversity, ensuring that meals are not only nutritious but also pleasant and easy to prepare. We hope to make the dietary journey as broad and satisfying as possible by include a variety of fruits, vegetables, lean proteins, whole grains, and healthy fats.

Furthermore, the 30-day meal plan provides a practical roadmap for adopting these nutritional modifications. It offers an organised approach to meal planning that can be tailored to individual preferences and nutritional requirements. Consistency with this regimen can result in noticeable improvements in health and daily functioning.

We invite readers to consider this cookbook as a starting point. Continuous learning, adaption, and interaction with healthcare professionals are required to effectively manage Huntington's disease. Embracing these dietary guidelines allows patients and carers to take proactive measures towards a better, more vibrant life despite the obstacles of Huntington's.

Remember that every meal provides an opportunity to nourish the body and support the brain. Let's make every bite count towards a higher quality of life.

THE END